Dr Sebi Cure for Diabetes

Proven and Simple Recipes Approved by Dr Sebi to Prevent and Reverse Diabetes, Using Herbs and Organic Food

Written By

Mark Smith

Table of Contents

INTRODUCTION

Thank you for purchasing this book!

Following these strategies to see results immediately:

Avoid food with preservatives and food colours. Our body has not been programmed to absorb such substances, and the body then absorbs them or retains them as fat, so they do not damage the liver. Chemicals create acids, such that the body neutralizes them either by generating cholesterols or blanching iron from the RBCs (leading to anaemia) or by extracting calcium from bones (osteoporosis).

Avoid artificial sweeteners. These sweeteners, which tend to be high in low fat, are potentially detrimental to the body. In addition, Saccharin, a primary ingredient in sweeteners, triggers cancer. Keep away from these things, therefore. Go for less healthy food, still a decent one.

Satiate your urges for a snack by eating vegetables or soaked nuts. Whenever we are thirsty, we still consume a little fast food. Establish a tradition of consuming fresh vegetables or almonds, even walnuts

Enjoy your reading!

SOUPS

Quick Broccoli Soup

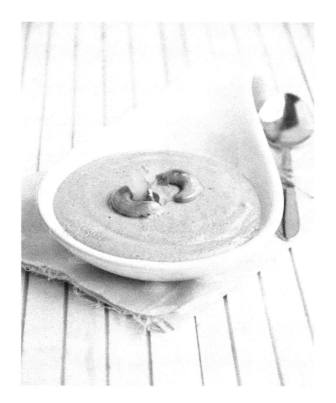

Preparation Time: 5 minutes

Cooking Time: 10 minutes

Servings: 6

Ingredients:

1 lb. broccoli, chopped

6 cups filtered alkaline water

1 onion, diced

2 tbsp. olive oil

Pepper Salt

Directions:

1. Add oil into the instant pot and set the pot on sauté mode.

2. Add the onion in olive oil and sauté until softened.

3. Add broccoli and water and stir well.

4. Cover pot with top and cook on manual high pressure for 3 minutes.

5. When finished, release pressure using the quick release, and then open the lid.

6. Blend the soup utilizing a submersion blender until smooth.

7. Season soup with pepper and salt.

8. Serve and enjoy.

Nutrition:

Calories 73

Fat 4.9 g

Carbohydrates 6.7 g

Protein 2.3 g

Sugar 2.1 g

Cholesterol 0 mg

Green Lentil Soup

Preparation Time: 10 minutes

Cooking Time: 30 minutes

Servings: 4

Ingredients:

1. ½ cups green lentils, rinsed

3 cups baby spinach

4 cups filtered alkaline water

2. tsp. Italian seasoning

3. tsp. fresh thyme

4. 14 oz. tomatoes, diced

   2 garlic cloves, minced

5. celery stalks, chopped

   1 carrot, chopped

   1 onion, chopped

6. Pepper

   i. Sea salt

Directions:

all ingredients except spinach into the direct pot and mix fine.

2. Cover pot with top and cook on manual high pressure for 18 minutes.

3. When finished, release pressure using the quick release, and then open the lid.

4. Add spinach and stir well.

5. Serve and enjoy.

Nutrition:

Calories 306

Fat 1.5 g

Carbohydrates 53.7 g

Sugar 6.4 g

Protein 21 g Cholesterol 1 mg

Squash Soup

Preparation Time: 10 minutes

Cooking Time: 40 minutes

Servings: 4

Ingredients:

3 lbs. butternut squash, peeled and cubed

1 tbsp. curry powder

1/2 cup unsweetened coconut milk

3 cups filtered alkaline water

2 garlic cloves, minced

1 large onion, minced

1 tsp. olive oil

Directions:

1. Add olive oil in the instant pot and set the pot on sauté mode.

2. onion and cook until tender, about 8 minutes.

3. Add curry powder and garlic and sauté for a minute.

4. Add butternut squash, water, and salt and stir well.

5. Cover pot with lid and cook on soup mode for 30 minutes.

6. When finished, release pressure naturally for 10 minutes, then release using the quick release, and then open the lid.

7. Blend the soup utilizing a submersion blender until smooth.

8. Add coconut milk and stir well.

9. Serve warm and enjoy.

Nutrition:

Calories 254

Fat 8.9 g

Carbohydrates 46.4 g

Sugar 10.1 g

Protein 4.8 g Cholesterol 0 mg

Tomato Soup

Preparation Time: 5 minutes

Cooking Time: 20 minutes

Servings: 4

Ingredients:

6 tomatoes, chopped

1 onion, diced

14 oz. coconut milk

1 tsp. turmeric

1 tsp. garlic, minced

1/4 cup cilantro, chopped

1/2 tsp. cayenne pepper

1 tsp. ginger, minced

1/2 tsp. sea salt

Directions:

all ingredients to the direct pot and mix fine.

2. Cover the instant pot with a lid and cook on manual high pressure for 5 minutes.

3. When finished, release pressure naturally for 10 minutes then release using the quick release.

4. Blend the soup utilizing a submersion blender until smooth.

5. Stir well and serve.

Nutrition:

Calories 81

Fat 3.5 g

Carbohydrates 11.6 g

Sugar 6.1 g

Protein 2.5 g

Cholesterol 0 mg

Basil Zucchini Soup

Preparation Time: 10 minutes

Cooking Time: 20 minutes

Servings: 4

Ingredients:

3 medium zucchinis, peeled and chopped

1/4 cup basil, chopped

1 large leek, chopped

3 cups filtered alkaline water

1 tbsp. lemon juice

3 tbsp. olive oil

1 tsp. sea salt

Directions:

1. Add 2 tbsp. oil into the pot and set the pot on sauté mode.

2. Add zucchini and sauté for 5 minutes.

3. Add basil and leeks and sauté for 2-3 minutes.

4.   lemon juice, water, and salt. Stir well.

5.   Cover pot with lid and cook on high pressure for 8 minutes.

6.   When finished, release pressure naturally, then open the lid.

7.   Blend the soup utilizing a submersion blender until smooth.

8.   Top with remaining olive oil and serve.

Nutrition:

Calories 157

Fat 11.9 g

Carbohydrates 8.9 g

Protein 5.8 g

Sugar 4 g

Cholesterol 0 mg

Summer Vegetable Soup

Preparation Time: 5 minutes

Cooking Time: 20 minutes

Servings: 10

Ingredients:

1/2 cup basil, chopped

2 bell peppers, seeded and sliced

1/ cup green beans, trimmed and cut into pieces

8 cups filtered alkaline water

1 medium summer squash, sliced

1 medium zucchini, sliced

2 large tomatoes, sliced 1 small eggplant, sliced

6 garlic cloves, smashed

1 medium onion, diced

Pepper Salt

Directions:

Combine all elements into the direct pot and mix fine.

2. Cover pot with lid and cook on soup mode for 10 minutes.

3. Release pressure using the quick release, then open the lid.

4. Blend the soup utilizing a submersion blender until smooth.

5. Serve and enjoy.

Nutrition:

Calories 84

Fat 1.6 g

Carbohydrates 12.8 g

Protein 6.1 g

Sugar 6.1 g

Cholesterol 0 mg

<u>Spicy Carrot Soup</u>

Preparation Time: 10 minutes

Cooking Time: 20 minutes

Servings: 6

Ingredients:

8 large carrots, peeled and chopped

1 1/2 cups filtered alkaline water

14 oz. coconut milk

3 garlic cloves, peeled

1 tbsp. red curry paste

1/4 cup olive oil

1 onion, chopped Salt

Directions:

1. Combine all elements into the direct pot and mix fine.
2. Cover the pot with a lid, select the manual, and set the timer for 15 minutes.
3. Release pressure naturally, then open the lid.

4. Blend the soup utilizing a submersion blender until smooth.

5. Serve and enjoy.

Nutrition:

Calories 267

Fat 22 g

Carbohydrates 13 g

Protein 4 g

Sugar 5 g Cholesterol 20 mg

Zucchini Soup

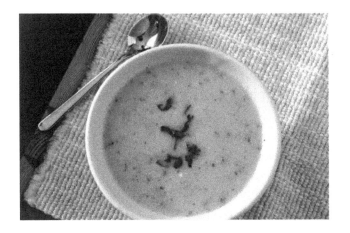

Preparation Time: 10 minutes

Cooking Time: 30 minutes

Servings: 10

Ingredients:

10 cups zucchini, chopped

32 oz. filtered alkaline water

13.5 oz. coconut milk

1 tbsp. Thai curry paste

Directions:

1. Combine all elements into the direct pot and mix fine.

2. Cover pot with lid and cook on manual high pressure for 10 minutes.

3. Release pressure using the quick release, then open the lid.

4. Use a blender to blend the soup until smooth.

5. Serve and enjoy.

Nutrition:

Calories 122

Fat 9.8 g

Carbohydrates 6.6 g

Protein 4.1 g

Sugar 3.6 g

Cholesterol 0 mg

Dill Celery Soup

Preparation Time: 10 minutes

Cooking Time: 30 minutes

Servings: 4

Ingredients:

6 cups celery stalk, chopped

2 cups filtered alkaline water

1 medium onion, chopped

1/2 tsp. dill

1 cup of coconut milk

1/4 tsp. sea salt

Directions:

1. Combine all elements into the direct pot and mix fine.

2. Cover pot with a lid and select soup mode; it takes 30 minutes.

3. Release pressure using the quick release, then open the lid carefully.

4. Blend the soup utilizing a submersion blender until smooth.

5. Stir well and serve.

Nutrition:

Calories 193

Fat 15.3 g

Carbohydrates 10.9 g

Protein 5.2 g

Sugar 5.6 g

Cholesterol 0 mg

SALADS

Beet Salad with Basil Dressing

Preparation Time: 10 minutes

Cooking Time: 0 minutes

Servings: 4

Ingredients:

Ingredients for the dressing:

¼ cup blackberries

¼ cup extra-virgin olive oil

Juice of 1 lemon

3 tablespoons minced fresh basil teaspoon poppy seeds A pinch of sea
salt
For the salad:
celery stalks, chopped

4 cooked beets, peeled and chopped

1 cup blackberries

1cups spring mix

Directions:

1. To make the dressing, mash the blackberries in a bowl. Whisk in the oil, lemon juice, basil, poppy seeds, and sea salt.

2. To make the salad: Add the celery, beets, blackberries, and spring mix to the bowl with the dressing.

3. Combine and serve.

Nutrition:

Calories: 192

Fat: 15g

Carbohydrates: 15g

Protein: 2g

Basic Salad with Olive Oil Dressing

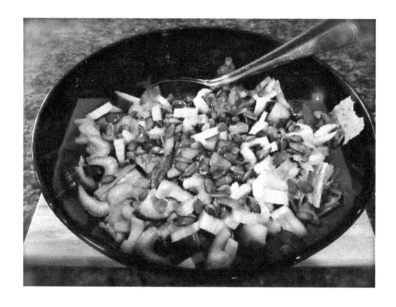

Preparation Time: 10 minutes

Cooking Time: 0 minute

Servings: 4

Ingredients:

1 cup coarsely chopped iceberg lettuce

1 cup coarsely chopped romaine lettuce

1 cup fresh baby spinach

1 large tomato, hulled and coarsely chopped

1 cup diced cucumber

2 tablespoons extra-virgin olive oil

¼ teaspoon of sea salt

Directions:

1. In a bowl, combine the spinach and lettuces. Add the tomato and cucumber.

2. Drizzle with oil and sprinkle with sea salt.

3. Mix and serve.

Nutrition:

Calories: 77

Fat: 4g

Carbohydrates: 3g

Protein: 1g

Spinach & Orange Salad with Oil Drizzle

Preparation Time: 10 minutes

Cooking Time: 0 minute

Servings: 4

Ingredients:

4 cups fresh baby spinach

1 blood orange, coarsely chopped

½ red onion, thinly sliced

½ shallot, finely chopped

2 tbsp. minced fennel fronds

Juice of 1 lemon

1 tbsp. extra-virgin olive oil A pinch of sea salt

Directions:

1. In a bowl, toss together the spinach, orange, red onion, shallot, and fennel fronds.

2. Add the lemon juice, oil, and sea salt.

3. Mix and serve.

Nutrition:

Calories: 79

Fat: 2g

Carbohydrates: 8g

Protein: 1g

Fruit Salad with Coconut-Lime Dressing

Preparation Time: 5 minutes

Cooking Time: 0 minutes

Servings: 4

Ingredients:

Ingredients for the dressing:

¼ cup full-fat canned coconut milk

1 tbsp. raw honey

Juice of ½ lime

A pinch of sea salt

For the salad

2 bananas, thinly sliced

2 mandarin oranges, segmented

½ cup strawberries, thinly sliced

½ cup raspberries

½ cup blueberries

Directions:

1. To make the dressing: whisk all the dressing ingredients in a bowl.

2. To make the salad: Add the salad ingredients in a bowl and mix.

3. Drizzle with the dressing and serve.

Nutrition:

Calories: 141

Fat: 3g

Carbohydrates: 30g

Protein: 2g

MAIN DISHES

Sweet and Sour Onions

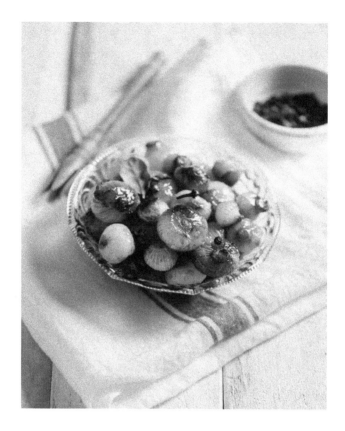

Preparation Time: 10 minutes

Cooking Time: 11 minutes

Servings: 4

Ingredients:

4 large onions, halved

2 garlic cloves, crushed

3 cups vegetable stock

1 ½ tablespoon balsamic vinegar

½ teaspoon Dijon mustard

1 tablespoon sugar

Directions:

1. Combine onions and garlic in a pan. Fry for 3 minutes, or till softened.

2. Pour stock, vinegar, Dijon mustard, and sugar. Bring to a boil.

3. Reduce heat. Cover and let the combination simmer for 10 minutes.

4. Get rid of from heat. Continue stirring until the liquid is reduced and the onions are brown. Serve.

Nutrition:

Calories 203

Total Fat 41.2 g

Saturated Fat 0.8 g

Cholesterol 0 mg

Sodium 861 mg

Total Carbs 29.5 g

Fiber 16.3 g

Sugar 29.3 g

Protein 19.2 g

Sautéed Apples and Onions

Preparation Time: 14 minutes

Cooking Time: 16 minutes

Servings: 3

Ingredients:

2 cups dry cider

1 large onion, halved

2 cups vegetable stock

4 apples, sliced into wedges

A pinch of salt

A pinch of pepper

Directions:

1. Combine cider and onion in a saucepan. Bring to a boil until the onions are cooked and liquid is almost gone.

2. Pour the stock and the apples. Season with salt and pepper. Stir occasionally. Cook for about 10 minutes or until the apples are tender but not mushy. Serve.

Nutrition:

Calories 343

Total Fat 51.2 g

Saturated Fat 0.8 g

Cholesterol 0 mg

Sodium 861 mg

Total Carbs 22.5 g

Fiber 6.3 g

Sugar 2.3 g

Protein 9.2 g

Zucchini Noodles with Portabella Mushrooms

Preparation Time: 14 minutes

Cooking Time: 16 minutes

Servings: 3

Ingredients:

1 zucchini, processed into spaghetti-like noodles

3 garlic cloves, minced

2 white onions, thinly sliced

1 thumb-sized ginger, julienned

1 lb. chicken thighs

1 lb. portabella mushrooms, sliced into thick slivers

2 cups chicken stock

3 cups of water

A pinch of sea salt, add more if needed

A pinch of black pepper, add more if needed

2 tsp. sesame oil

4 tbsp. coconut oil, divided

¼ cup fresh chives, minced, for garnish **Directions:**

1. Pour 2 tablespoons of coconut oil into a large saucepan. Fry mushroom slivers in batches for 5 minutes or until seared brown. Set aside. Transfer these to a plate.

2. Sauté the onion, garlic, and ginger for 3 minutes or until tender.
   Add in chicken thighs, cooked mushrooms, chicken stock, water, salt, and pepper stir mixture well. Bring to a boil.

3. Decrease gradually the heat and allow simmering for 20 minutes or until the chicken is forking tender. Tip in sesame oil.

4. Serve by placing an equal amount of zucchini noodles into bowls. Ladle soup and garnish with chives.

Nutrition:

Calories 163

Total Fat 4.2 g

Saturated Fat 0.8 g

Cholesterol 0 mg

Sodium 861 mg

Total Carbs 22.5 g

Fiber 6.3 g

Sugar 2.3 g

Protein 9.2 g

Grilled Tempeh with Pineapple

Preparation Time: 12 minutes

Cooking Time: 16 minutes

Servings: 3

Ingredients:

10 oz. tempeh, sliced

1 red bell pepper, quartered

1/4 pineapple, sliced into rings

6 oz. green beans

1 tbsp. coconut aminos

2 1/2 tbsp. orange juice, freshly squeeze

1 1/2 tbsp. lemon juice, freshly squeezed

1 tbsp. extra virgin olive oil

1/4 cup hoisin sauce

Directions:

1. Blend the olive oil, orange and lemon juices, coconut aminos or soy sauce, and hoisin sauce in a bowl. Add the diced tempeh and set aside.

2. Heat up the grill or place a grill pan over medium-high flame. Once hot, lift the marinated tempeh from the bowl with a pair of tongs and transfer them to the grill or pan.

3. Grill for 2 to 3 minutes, or until browned all over.

4. Grill the sliced pineapples alongside the tempeh, then transfer them directly onto the serving platter.

5. Place the grilled tempeh beside the grilled pineapple and cover with aluminium foil to keep warm.

6. Meanwhile, place the green beans and bell peppers in a bowl and add just enough of the marinade to coat.

7. Prepare the grill pan and add the vegetables. Grill until fork tender and slightly charred.

8. Transfer the grilled vegetables to the serving platter and arrange artfully with the tempeh and pineapple. Serve at once.

Nutrition:

Calories 163

Total Fat 4.2 g

Saturated Fat 0.8 g

Cholesterol 0 mg

Sodium 861 mg

Total Carbs 22.5 g

Fiber 6.3 g

Sugar 2.3 g

Protein 9.2 g

Courgettes in Cider Sauce

Preparation Time: 13 minutes

Cooking Time: 17 minutes

Servings: 3

Ingredients:

2 cups baby courgettes

3 tablespoons vegetable stock

2 tablespoons apple cider vinegar

1 tablespoon light brown sugar

4 spring onions, finely sliced

1 piece of fresh ginger root, grated

1teaspoon of corn flour

5   teaspoons of water

Directions:

6   Bring a pan with salted water to a boil.

7   Add courgettes. Bring to a boil for 5 minutes.

8   Meanwhile, in a pan, combine vegetable stock, apple cider vinegar, brown sugar, onions, ginger root, lemon juice and rind, and

orange juice and rind. Take to a boil. Lower the heat and allow simmering for 3 minutes.

9   Mix the corn flour with water. Stir well. Pour into the sauce.

10   Continue stirring until the sauce thickens.

11   Drain courgettes. Transfer to the serving dish. Spoon over the sauce. Toss to coat courgettes. Serve.

Nutrition:

Calories 173

Total Fat 9.2 g

Saturated Fat 0.8 g

Cholesterol 0 mg

Sodium 861 mg

Total Carbs 22.5 g

Fiber 6.3 g

Sugar 2.3 g

Protein 9.2 g

Baked Mixed Mushrooms

Preparation Time: 8 minutes

Cooking Time: 20 minutes

Servings: 3

Ingredients:

2 cups mixed wild mushrooms

1 cup chestnut mushrooms

2 cups dried porcini

2 shallots

4 garlic cloves

3 cups raw pecans

½ bunch fresh thyme

1 bunch flat-leaf parsley

2 tablespoons olive oil

2 fresh bay leaves

1 ½ cups stale bread

Directions:

1. Remove skin and finely chop garlic and shallots. Roughly chop the wild mushrooms and chestnut mushrooms. Pick the leaves of the thyme and tear the bread into small pieces. Put inside the pressure cooker.

2. Place the pecans and roughly chop the nuts. Pick the parsley leaves and roughly chop.

3. Place the porcini in a bowl then add 300ml of boiling water. Set aside until needed.

4. Heat oil in the pressure cooker. Add the garlic and shallots. Cook for 3 minutes while stirring occasionally.

5. Drain porcini and reserve the liquid. Add the porcini into the pressure cooker together with the wild mushrooms and chestnut mushrooms. Add the bay leaves and thyme.

6. Position the lid and lock in place. Put to high heat and bring to high pressure. Adjust heat to stabilize. Cook for 10 minutes. Adjust taste if necessary.

7. Transfer the mushroom mixture into a bowl and set aside to cool completely.

8. Once the mushrooms are completely cool, add the bread, pecans, a pinch of black pepper and sea salt, and half of the

reserved liquid into the bowl. Mix well. Add more reserved liquid if the mixture seems dry.

9. Add more than half of the parsley into the bowl and stir. Transfer the mixture into a 20cm x 25cm lightly greased baking dish and cover with tin foil.

10. Bake in the oven for 35 minutes. Then, get rid of the foil and cook for another 10 minutes. Once done, sprinkle the remaining parsley on top and serve with bread or crackers. Serve.

Nutrition:

Calories 343

Total Fat 4.2 g

Saturated Fat 0.8 g

Cholesterol 0 mg

Sodium 861 mg

Total Carbs 22.5 g

Fiber 6.3 g

Sugar 2.3 g

Protein 9.2 g

Spiced Okra

Preparation Time: 14 minutes

Cooking Time: 16 minutes

Servings: 3

Ingredients:

2 cups okra

¼ teaspoon stevia

1 teaspoon chilli powder

½ teaspoon ground turmeric

1 tablespoon ground coriander

2 tablespoons fresh coriander, chopped

1 tablespoon ground cumin

¼ teaspoon salt

1 tablespoon desiccated coconut

3 tablespoons vegetable oil

½ teaspoon black mustard seeds

½ teaspoon cumin seeds

Fresh tomatoes, to garnish

Directions:

1. Trim the okra. Wash and dry.

2. Combine stevia, chilli powder, turmeric, ground coriander, fresh coriander, cumin, salt, and desiccated coconut in a bowl.

3. Heat the oil in a pan. Cook mustard and cumin seeds for 3 minutes. Stir continuously. Add okra. Tip in the spice mixture. Cook on low heat for 8 minutes.

4. Transfer to a serving dish. Garnish with fresh tomatoes.

Nutrition:

Calories 163

Total Fat 4.2 g

Saturated Fat 0.8 g

Cholesterol 0 mg

Sodium 861 mg

Total Carbs 22.5 g

Fiber 6.3 g

Sugar 2.3 g

Protein 9.2 g

SAUCES

Fragrant Tomato Sauce

Preparation Time: 14 minutes

Cooking Time: 16 minutes

Servings: 3

Ingredients:

5 Roma tomatoes

1 pinch of basil

1 teaspoon of oregano

1 teaspoon of onion powder

2 teaspoon of minced onion

2 teaspoon agave syrup

1 teaspoon of pure sea salt

2 tablespoons of grape seed oil

Directions:

1. Make an X cut on the lowermost of the Roma tomatoes and place them into a pot of hot water for just 1 minute. Take away the tomatoes from the water using a spoon and shock them, placing them in cold water for 30 seconds. Take them out and immediately peel with your fingers or a knife. Put all

the ingredients into a mixer or a food processor and blend for 1 minute until smooth.

Serve and enjoy your fragrant tomato sauce.

Nutrition:

Calories: 20

Carbohydrates: 2 g

Protein: 1g

Guacamole

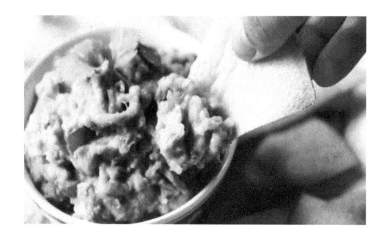

Preparation Time: 14 minutes

Cooking Time: 16 minutes

Servings: 3

Ingredients:

1 minced Roma tomato

2 avocados

1/2 cup of chopped cilantro

1/2 cup of minced red onion

1/2 teaspoon of cayenne powder

1/2 teaspoon of onion powder

1/2 teaspoon of pure sea salt Juice from ½ lime

Directions:

1. Cut the avocados in half, peel, and remove the seeds. Slice into tiny pieces and put them in a medium bowl. Add all other ingredients, excluding the Roma tomato, to the bowl. Using a masher, mix together until becomes smooth. Add the minced Roma tomatoes to the mixture and mix well.

2. Serve and enjoy your delicious guacamole!

Nutrition:

Calories: 12

Fat: 1 g

Garlic Sauce

Preparation Time: 14 minutes

Cooking Time: 16 minutes

Servings: 3

Ingredients:

1/4 cup of diced shallots

1 tablespoon of onion powder

1/4 teaspoon of dill

1/2 teaspoon of ginger

1/2 teaspoon of pure sea salt

1 cup of grapeseed oil

Directions:

1. Find a glass jar with a lid. Put all ingredients for the sauce in the jar and shake them well. Place the sauce mixture in the refrigerator for at least 1 hour. Serve and enjoy your "garlic" sauce!

Nutrition:

Calories: 48

Carbohydrates: 2 g

Fat: 4 g

Pesto Saucy Cream Recipe

Preparation Time: 14 minutes

Cooking Time: 16 minutes

Servings: 3

Ingredients:

1 small avocado (Hass)

1 cup walnuts

3 tablespoons sour orange or lime

1/8 teaspoon basil

1/4 teaspoon onion powder

1/4 teaspoon cayenne pepper

1 teaspoon spring water

Directions:

1. Make a slit with a knife lengthwise around the avocado. Split open the avocado into two. Then using your heavy knife carefully, hit down the avocado seed, turn and pull out the seed. Scoop out the avocado meat and remove the skin. Then, add all of the ingredients to your blender and blend

until all of the ingredients are thoroughly mixed and becomes smooth.

Nutrition:

Calories: 65

Carbohydrates: 4 g

Fat: 5 g

Protein: 3 g

SPECIAL
INGREDIENTS

Dill Cucumber Dressing

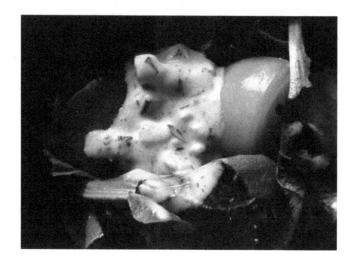

Preparation Time: 5 minutes

Cooking Time: 10 minutes

Servings: 1/2 cups **Ingredients:**

1 teaspoon of fresh dill*

1 cup of quartered cucumbers

1/2 teaspoon of onion powder

2 teaspoons of agave syrup

1 tablespoon of lime juice

1/4 cup of Avocado oil

Directions:

1. Prepare and place all ingredients into the blender.

2. Blend for one minute until smooth.

3. Add it to a salad and enjoy your dill cucumber dressing!

Nutrition:

Calories: 60

Carbohydrates: 3 g

Fat: 5

Homemade Walnut Milk

Preparation Time: 15 minutes

Cooking Time: Minimum 8 hours

Servings: 4 cups **Ingredients:**

1 cup of raw walnuts

1/8 teaspoon of pure sea salt

3 cups of spring water + extra for soaking

Directions:

1. Put raw walnuts in a small pot and cover them with three inches of water.

2. Soak the walnuts for at least eight hours.

3. Drain and rinse the walnuts with cold water.

4. Add the soaked walnuts, pure sea salt, and three cups of spring water to a blender.

5. Mix well until smooth.

6. Strain it if you need to.

7. Enjoy your homemade walnut milk!

Nutrition:

Calories: 200

Carbohydrate: 3.89 gr

Sugar: 1 g

Fiber: 2 g

Protein: 5 g

Fat: 20

Aquafaba

Preparation Time: 15 minutes

Cooking Time: 2 Hours 30 Minutes

Servings: 2-4 Cups **Ingredients:**

1 bag of garbanzo beans

1 teaspoon of pure sea salt

5   cups of spring water + extra for soaking

Directions:

1. Place garbanzo beans in a large pot, add spring water and pure sea salt. Bring to a rolling boil.

2. Remove from the heat and leave to soak kindly for 30 to 40 minutes.

3. Strain garbanzo beans and add 6 cups of spring water.

4. Boil for 1 hour and 30 minutes on medium heat.

5. Strain the garbanzo beans. This strained water is Aquafaba.

6. Pour Aquafaba into a glass jar with a lid and place it into the refrigerator.

7. After cooling, Aquafaba becomes thicker. If it is too liquid, repeatedly boil for 10-20 minutes.

Useful tips:

Aquafaba is a good alternative for an egg: 2 tablespoons of Aquafaba = 1 egg white 3 tablespoons of Aquafaba = 1 egg.

Nutrition:

Calories: 46

Carbs: 8 g

Fiber: 2 g

Protein: 3 g

SNACKS & BREAD

Potato Chips

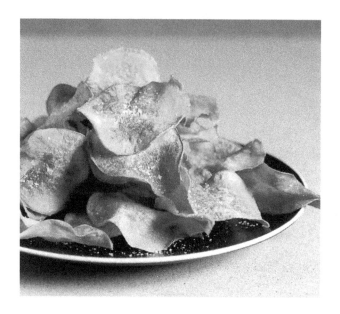

Preparation Time: 10 minutes

Cooking Time: 20 minutes

Servings: 4

Ingredients:

1 tablespoon vegetable oil 1 potato, sliced paper-thin Sea salt, to taste

Directions:

1. Toss potato with oil and sea salt.

2. Spread the slices in a baking dish in a single layer.

3. Cook in a microwave for 5 minutes until golden brown.

4. Serve.

Nutrition:

Calories 80

Total Fat 3.5 g

Saturated Fat 0.1 g

Cholesterol 320 mg

Sodium 350 mg

Total Carbs 11.6 g

Fiber 0.7 g

Sugar 0.7 g

Protein 1.2 g

Zucchini Pepper Chips

Preparation Time: 10 minutes

Cooking Time: 15 minutes

Servings: 04 **Ingredients:**

1 2/3 cups vegetable oil

1 teaspoon garlic powder 1 teaspoon onion powder

1/2 teaspoon black pepper

3 tablespoons crushed red pepper flakes

2 zucchinis, thinly sliced

Directions:

1. Mix oil with all the spices in a bowl.

2. Add zucchini slices and mix well.

3. Transfer the mixture to a Ziplock bag and seal it.

4. Refrigerate for 10 minutes.

5. Spread the zucchini slices on a greased baking sheet. 6. Bake for 15 minutes 7. Serve.

Nutrition:

Calories 172

Total Fat 11.1 g

Saturated Fat 5.8 g

Cholesterol 610 mg

Sodium 749 mg

Total Carbs 19.9 g

Fiber 0.2 g

Sugar 0.2 g

Protein 13.5 g

Apple Chips

Preparation Time: 5 minutes

Cooking Time: 45 minutes

Servings: 4

Ingredients:

2 Golden Delicious apples, cored and thinly sliced

1 1/2 teaspoons white sugar

1/2 teaspoon ground cinnamon

Directions:

1. Set your oven to 225 degrees F.

2. Place apple slices on a baking sheet.

3. Sprinkle sugar and cinnamon over apple slices.

4. Bake for 45 minutes.

5. Serve

Nutrition:

Calories 127

Total Fat 3.5 g

Saturated Fat 0.5 g

Cholesterol 162 mg

Sodium 142 mg

Total Carbs 33.6g

Fiber 0.4 g

Sugar 0.5 g

Protein 4.5 g

Kale Crisps

Preparation Time: 10 minutes

Cooking Time: 10 minutes

Servings: 04

Ingredients:

1 bunch kale, remove the stems, leaves torn into even pieces

1 tablespoon of olive oil

1 teaspoon of sea salt

Directions:

1. Set your oven to 350 degrees F. Layer a baking sheet with parchment paper.

2. Spread the kale leaves on a paper towel to absorb all the moisture.

3. Toss the leaves with sea salt and olive oil.

4. Kindly spread them on the baking sheet and bake for 10 minutes.

5. Serve.

Nutrition:

Calories 113

Total Fat 7.5 g

Saturated Fat 1.1 g

Cholesterol 20 mg

Sodium 97 mg

Total Carbs 1.4 g

Fiber 0 g

Sugar 0 g

Protein 1.1g

Carrot Chips

Preparation Time: 5 minutes

Cooking Time: 12 minutes

Servings: 4

Ingredients:

4 carrots, washed, peeled and sliced

2 teaspoons of extra-virgin olive oil

1/4 teaspoon of sea salt

Directions:

1. Set your oven to 350 degrees F.
2. Toss carrots with salt and olive oil.
3. Spread the slices into two baking sheets in a single layer.
4. Bake for 6 minutes on the upper and lower rack of the oven.
5. Switch the baking racks and bake for another 6 minutes.
6. Serve.

Nutrition:

Calories 153

Total Fat 7.5 g

Saturated Fat 1.1 g

Cholesterol 20 mg

Sodium 97 mg

Total Carbs 20.4 g

Fiber 0 g

Sugar 0 g

Protein 3.1g

Pita Chips

Preparation Time: 5 minutes

Cooking Time: 12 minutes

Servings: 4

Ingredients:

12 pita bread pockets, sliced into triangles

1/2 cup olive oil

1/2 teaspoon ground black pepper

1 teaspoon of garlic salt 1/2 teaspoon dried basil

1 teaspoon dried chervil

Directions:

1. Set your oven to 400 degrees F.

2. Toss pita with all the remaining ingredients in a bowl.

3. Spread the seasoned triangles on a baking sheet.

4. Bake for 7 minutes until golden brown.

5. Serve with your favourite hummus.

Nutrition:

Calories 201

Total Fat 5.5 g

Saturated Fat 2.1 g

Cholesterol 10 mg

Sodium 597 mg

Total Carbs 2.4 g

Fiber 0 g

Sugar 0 g

Protein 3.1g

Sweet Potato Chips

Preparation Time: 5 minutes

Cooking Time: 5 minutes

Servings: 4

Ingredients:

1   sweet potato, thinly sliced

2   teaspoons olive oil, or as needed

3   Coarse sea salt, to taste

Directions:

1. Toss sweet potato with oil and salt.

2. Spread the slices in a baking dish in a single layer.

3. Cook in a microwave for 5 minutes until golden brown.

4. Serve.

Nutrition:

Calories 213

Total Fat 8.5 g

Saturated Fat 3.1 g
Cholesterol 120 mg

Sodium 497 mg

Total Carbs 21.4 g

Fiber 0 g

Sugar 0 g

Protein 0.1g

DESSERTS

Blueberry Muffins

Preparation Time: 5 minutes

Cooking Time: 1 Hour

Servings: 3

Ingredients:

1/2 cup of blueberries

3/4 cup of teff flour

3/4 cup of spelt flour

1/3 cup of agave syrup

1/2 teaspoon of pure sea salt

1 cup of coconut milk

1/4 cup of sea moss gel (optional, check information) Grape Seed Oil

Directions:

1. Preheat your oven to 365 degrees Fahrenheit.

2. Grease or line 6 standard muffin cups.

3. Add Teff, Spelt flour, Pure Sea Salt, Coconut Milk, Sea Moss Gel, and Agave Syrup to a large bowl. Mix them together.

4. Add Blueberries to the mixture and mix well.

5. Divide muffin batter among the 6 muffin cups.

6. Bake for 30 minutes until golden brown.

7. Serve and enjoy your Blueberry Muffins!

Nutrition:

Calories: 65

Fat: 0.7 g

Carbohydrates: 12 g

Protein: 1.4 g

Fiber: 5 g

Banana Strawberry Ice Cream

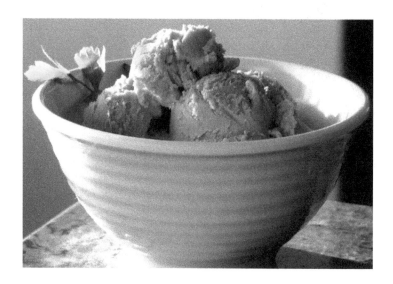

Preparation Time: 5 minutes

Cooking Time: 4 hours

Servings: 5

Ingredients:

1 cup of strawberry*

5 quartered baby bananas*

1/2 avocado, chopped

1 tablespoon of agave syrup

1/4 cup of homemade walnut milk

Directions:

1. Mix ingredients into the blender and blend them well.

2. Taste. If it is too thick, add extra milk or agave syrup if you want it sweeter.

3. Put in a container with a lid and allow to freeze for at least 5 to 6 hours.

4. Serve it and enjoy your banana strawberry ice cream!

Nutrition:

Calories: 200

Fat: 0.5 g

Carbohydrates: 44 g

Homemade Whipped Cream

Preparation Time: 5 minutes

Cooking Time: 10 minutes

Servings: 1 Cup **Ingredients:**

1 cup of Aquafaba

1/4 cup of agave syrup

Directions:

1. Add agave syrup and Aquafaba into a bowl.

2. Mix at high speed around 5 minutes with a stand mixer or 10 to 15 minutes with a hand mixer.

3. Serve and enjoy your homemade whipped cream!

Nutrition:

Calories: 21

Fat: 0g

Sodium: 0.3g

Carbohydrates: 5.3g

Fiber: 0g

Sugars: 4.7g

Protein: 0g

"Chocolate" Pudding

Preparation Time: 5 minutes

Cooking Time: 20 minutes

Servings: 4

Ingredients:

1 to 2 cups of black sapote

1/4 cup of agave syrup

1/2 cup of soaked Brazil nuts (overnight or for at least 3 hours)

1 tablespoon of hemp seeds

 1/2 cup of spring water

Directions:

1. Cut 1 to 2 cups of black sapote in half.

2. Remove all seeds. You should have 1 full cup of de-seeded fruit.

3. Mix all ingredients into a blender and blend until smooth.

4. Serve and enjoy your "chocolate" pudding!

Nutrition:

Calories: 134

Fat: 0.5 g

Carbohydrates: 15 g

Protein: 2.5 g

Fiber: 10 g

Banana Nut Muffins

Preparation Time: 5 minutes

Cooking Time: 1 Hour

Servings: 6

Ingredients:

Dry ingredients:

1 1/2 cups of spelt or teff flour

1/2 teaspoon of pure sea salt

3/4 cup of date syrup Wet ingredients:

2 medium blended burro bananas

¼ cup of grape seed oil

¾ cup of homemade walnut milk (see recipe)*

1 tablespoon of key lime juice
Filling ingredients:

½ cup of chopped walnuts (plus extra for decorating)

 1 chopped burro banana

Directions:

1. Preheat your oven to 400 degrees Fahrenheit.

2. Take a muffin tray and grease 12 cups or line with cupcake liners.

3. Put all dry ingredients in a large bowl and mix them thoroughly.

4. Add all wet ingredients to a separate, smaller bowl and mix well with blended bananas.

5. Mix ingredients from the two bowls in one large container. Be careful not to over mix.

6. Add the filling ingredients and fold in gently.

7. Pour muffin batter into the 12 prepared muffin cups and garnish with a couple of Walnuts.

8. Bake it for 22 to 26 minutes until golden brown.

9. Allow cooling for 10 minutes.

10. Serve and enjoy your banana nut muffins!

Nutrition:

Calories: 150

Fat: 10 g

Carbohydrates: 30 g

Protein: 2.4 g

Fiber: 2 g

Mango Nut Cheesecake

Cooking Time: 4 Hour 30 Minutes

Servings: 8 Servings

Ingredients:

Filling:

2 cups of Brazil nuts

5 to 6 dates

1 tablespoon of sea moss gel (check information)

1/4 cup of agave syrup

1/4 teaspoon of pure sea salt

2 tablespoons of lime juice

1 1/2 cups of homemade walnut milk (see recipe)*

Crust:

1 1/2 cups of quartered dates

1/4 cup of agave syrup

1 1/2 cups of coconut flakes

1/4 teaspoon of pure sea salt Toppings:

Sliced mango

Sliced strawberries

Directions:

Put all crust ingredients in a food processor and blend for 30 seconds.

With parchment paper, cover a baking form and spread out the blended crust ingredients.

Put sliced mango across the crust and freeze for 10 minutes.

Mix all filling ingredients using a blender until it becomes smooth. Pour the filling above the crust, cover with foil or parchment paper, and let it stand for about 3 to 4 hours in the refrigerator.

Take out from the baking form and garnish with toppings. Serve and enjoy your mango nut cheesecake!

Blackberry Jam

Preparation Time: 5 minutes

Cooking Time: 4 hours 30 minutes

Servings: 1 cup **Ingredients:**

3/4 cup of blackberries

1 tablespoon of key lime juice

3 tablespoons of agave syrup

¼ cup of sea moss gel + extra 2 tablespoons (check information)

Directions:

1. Put rinsed blackberries into a medium pot and cook on medium heat.

2. Stir blackberries until liquid appears.

3. Once berries soften, use your immersion blender to chop up any large pieces. If you don't have a blender put the mixture in a food processor, mix it well, then return to the pot.

4. Add sea moss gel, key lime juice, and agave syrup to the blended mixture. Boil on medium heat and stir well until it becomes thick.

5. Remove from the heat and leave it to cool for 10 minutes.

6. Serve it with bread pieces or the Flatbread (see recipe).

7. Enjoy your blackberry jam!

Nutrition:

Calories: 43

Fat: 0.5 g

Carbohydrates: 13 g

Blackberry Bars

Preparation Time: 5 minutes

Cooking Time: 1 hour 20 minutes

Servings: 4

Ingredients:

3 burro bananas or 4 baby bananas

1 cup of spelt flour

2 cups of quinoa flakes

1/4 cup of agave syrup

1/4 teaspoon of pure sea salt

1/2 cup of grape seed oil

1 cup of prepared blackberry jam

Directions:

1 Preheat your oven to 350 degrees Fahrenheit.

2 Remove the skin of the bananas and mash with a fork in a large bowl.

3 Combine agave syrup and grape seed oil with the blend and mix well.

4 Add spelt flour and quinoa flakes. Knead the dough until it becomes sticky to your fingers.

5 Cover a 9x9-inch baking pan with parchment paper.

6 Take 2/3 of the dough and smooth it out over the parchment pan with your fingers.

7 Spread blackberry jam over the dough.

8 Crumble the remaining dough and sprinkle on the top.

9 Bake for 20 minutes.

10 Remove from the oven and let it cool for at 10 to 15 minutes.

11 Cut into small pieces.

12 Serve and enjoy your blackberry bars!

Nutrition:

Calories: 43

Fat: 0.5 g

Carbohydrates: 10 g

Protein: 1.4 g

Fiber: 5 g

SMOOTHIES

Multiple Berries Smoothie

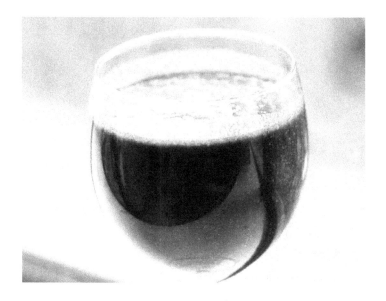

Preparation Time: 15 minutes

Cooking Time: 0

Servings: 1

Ingredients:

A quarter cupful of blueberries

A quarter cupful of strawberries

A quarter cupful of raspberries

One large banana (peeled and sliced)

Agave syrup as desired A half cupful of water

Directions:

1. Transfer the water into the blender.

2. Add the remaining recipes and blend until smooth.

3. I really love this smoothie because it is very sweet without adding sugar and the colour is also inviting.

Nutrition:

Calories: 210

Carbohydrates: 55 g

Sodium: 20 mg

Dandelion Avocado Smoothie

Preparation Time: 15 minutes

Cooking Time: 0

Servings: 1

Ingredients:

One cup of dandelion

One orange (juiced)

Coconut water

One avocado

One key lime (juice)

Directions:

1. In a high-speed blend all ingredients until smooth.

Nutrition:

Calories: 160

Fat: 15 grams

Carbohydrates: 9 grams

Protein: 2 grams

Amaranth Greens and Avocado Smoothie

Preparation Time: 15 minutes

Cooking Time: 0

Servings: 1

Ingredients:

One key lime (juice)

Two sliced apples (seeded)

Half avocado

Two cups of amaranth greens

Two cups of watercress One cup of water

Directions:

1. Add the whole recipes together and transfer them into the blender. Blend thoroughly until smooth.

Nutrition:

Calories: 160

Fat: 15 grams

Carbohydrates: 9 grams

Protein: 2 grams

Lettuce, Orange and Banana Smoothie

Preparation Time: 15 minutes

Cooking Time: 0

Servings: 1

Ingredients:

One and a half cupsful of fresh lettuce

One large banana

One cup of mixed berries of your choice One juiced orange

Directions:

1. First, add the orange juice to your blender.

2. Add the remaining recipes and blend thoroughly.

3. Enjoy the rest of your day.

Nutrition:

Calories: 252.1

Protein: 4.1 g

Delicious Elderberry Smoothie

Preparation Time: 15 minutes

Cooking Time: 0

Servings: 1

Ingredients:

One cupful of elderberry

One cupful of cucumber

One large apple

A quarter cupful of water

Directions:

1. Add the whole recipes together into a blender. Grind very well until they are uniformly smooth and enjoy.

Nutrition:

Calories: 106

Carbohydrates: 26.68

Peaches Zucchini Smoothie

Preparation Time: 15 minutes

Cooking Time: 0

Servings: 1

Ingredients:

A half cupful of squash

A half cupful of peaches

A quarter cupful of coconut water A half cupful of Zucchini

Directions:

1. Add the whole recipes together into a blender and blend until smooth and serve.

Nutrition:

55 Calories

0g Fat

2g Protein

10mg Sodium

14g Carbohydrate

2g Fiber

Ginger Orange and Strawberry Smoothie

Preparation Time: 15 minutes

Cooking Time: 0

Servings: 1

Ingredients:

One cup of strawberry

One large orange (juice)

One large banana

Quarter small sized ginger (peeled and sliced)

Directions:

1. Transfer the orange juice to a clean blender.

2. Add the remaining recipes and blend thoroughly until smooth.

3. Enjoy. Wow! You have ended the 9th day of your weight loss and detox journey.

Nutrition:

32 Calories

0.3g Fat

2g Protein

10mg Sodium

14g Carbohydrate

Water

2g Fiber

Kale Parsley and Chia Seeds Detox Smoothie

Preparation Time: 15 minutes

Cooking Time: 0

Servings: 1

Ingredients:

Three tbsp. chia seeds (grounded)

One cupful of water

One sliced banana

One pear (chopped)

One cupful of organic kale

One cupful of parsley

Two tbsp. of lemon juice A dash of cinnamon **Directions:**

1. Add the whole recipes together into a blender and pour the water before blending. Blend at high speed until smooth and enjoy. You may or may not place it in the refrigerator, depending on how hot or cold the weather appears.

Nutrition:

75 Calories

1g Fat

5g Protein

10g Fiber

CONCLUSION

Thank you for reading all this book!

It is prudent to attempt Dr. Sebi's Directions for 30 days if you don't completely receive another dietary system. Connect with for a month and see the upgrades. Following a month, you should change to this eating regimen altogether.

Dr. Sebi's diet advances eating entire, natural, plant-based food. Numerous people have used to cause a noteworthy change in their wellbeing. They are perfect in moving from acidic to soluble. You can similarly utilize them for occasionally keeping up your body framework and improving your wellbeing.

You have already taken a step towards your improvement.

Best wishes!

CPSIA information can be obtained
at www.ICGtesting.com
Printed in the USA
BVHW090451120521
607041BV00004B/1027